This book was compiled by Daniel Melehi
with the A.I assistance of Inventabot

<u>Dedication</u>

I hope this helps all of my wonderful
readers achieve all their goals in their
business. And I would like to thank my
wonderful wife for all of her continued
support in all my ventures.

©Daniel Melehi

May 7 2023

Contents

Chapter 1: Understanding Depression

Depression is a complex and serious mental health condition that affects millions of people worldwide. It is not just feeling sad or low but rather a persistent feeling of hopelessness, helplessness, and a lack of interest in activities that were once enjoyed.

SUBCHAPTER 1.1: CAUSES OF DEPRESSION

The causes of depression can be diverse and complex, and it varies from person to person. One of the leading causes of depression is a chemical imbalance in the brain, which affects the way we feel. The other factors that can lead to depression include genetics, certain medications, physical illnesses, significant life changes or events, and negative thought patterns.

SUBCHAPTER 1.2: TYPES OF DEPRESSION

There are several types of depression, and each one differs in symptoms, severity, and duration. Some of the most common types of depression are:

Major Depressive Disorder

It is the most prevalent type of depression and is characterized by a persistent low mood and loss of interest or pleasure in activities.

Persistent Depressive Disorder

It is a type of depression that lasts for a more extended period, typically two years or more, and can affect daily life.

Bipolar Disorder

It is a type of depression that is characterized by alternating periods of elevated or high moods (mania) and extremely low moods (depression).

Postpartum Depression

It is a type of depression that some women experience after giving birth.

Seasonal Affective Disorder

It is a type of depression that occurs during the winter months when there is less sunlight. It is crucial to recognize the signs and symptoms of depression early on, so it can be treated effectively. The next chapter will explore how to recognize depression.

SUBCHAPTER 1.1: CAUSES OF DEPRESSION

Depression is a complex mental illness that can be caused by various factors. The causes of depression can be classified into three major categories, including biological, psychological, and environmental factors.

Biological Factors:

Research suggests that an imbalance of certain chemicals in the brain, such as serotonin and dopamine, can contribute to depression. Genetics may also be a factor, as studies have shown that depression can run in families. Additionally, certain medical conditions such as thyroid disorders, chronic pain, and substance abuse can increase the risk of depression.

Psychological Factors:

Negative thinking patterns and stress can also trigger depression. People who have experienced trauma or significant life changes, such as the loss of a loved one or a job, are at a higher risk of developing depression. Additionally, people who struggle with self-esteem, have difficulty coping with emotions, or have a history of anxiety or other mental health issues may also be more vulnerable.

Environmental Factors:

Environmental factors such as social isolation, financial issues, and a lack of social support can contribute to depression. Living in stressful or unsafe environments can also increase the risk. Additionally, exposure to discrimination, racism, and abuse can contribute to depression and other mental health issues. Understanding the causes of depression can help individuals and their loved ones recognize the risk factors and seek appropriate support. It is important to note that depression is a treatable illness, and seeking help is a courageous step towards healing and recovery.

SUBCHAPTER 1.2: TYPES OF DEPRESSION

Depression can manifest in different ways, which is why it is classified into different types. Knowing these types can help with identifying the symptoms and seeking appropriate treatment. Here are some of the most common types of depression:

Major Depression

Also known as clinical depression, major depression is characterized by persistent feelings of sadness, hopelessness, loss of interest in activities, and low energy levels. These symptoms can last for weeks or months and can interfere with daily life. Major depression can be caused by various factors such as genetics, life events, and chemical imbalances in the brain.

Dysthymia

Dysthymia is a milder form of depression that lasts for two years or more. It is characterized by feelings of sadness, lack of motivation, and irritability. Dysthymia can impact a person's ability to function normally and it can often go undiagnosed.

Bipolar Disorder

Bipolar disorder, also known as manic depression, is a type of mood disorder that is characterized by mood swings between highs (mania) and lows (depression). During manic episodes, a person may experience elevated moods, exaggerated self-confidence, and risky behavior. During depressive episodes, they may experience feelings of sadness, hopelessness, and low energy. Bipolar disorder can be treated with medication and therapy.

Seasonal Affective Disorder (SAD)

SAD is a type of depression that is related to the change in seasons. It usually occurs during the fall and winter months when there is less sunlight. Symptoms of SAD include feelings of hopelessness, low energy levels, and changes in appetite. Treatment may involve light therapy, medication, and therapy.

Postpartum Depression

Postpartum depression is a type of depression that affects women after giving birth. It is caused by hormonal changes, physical changes, and the stress of caring for a newborn. Symptoms include feelings of sadness, anxiety, and loss of interest in activities. Treatment may involve therapy and medication.

Psychotic Depression

Psychotic depression is a type of depression that includes symptoms of psychosis, such as delusions and hallucinations. It can be caused by genetics, chemical imbalances in the brain, and substance abuse. It can be treated with medication and therapy. Understanding the different types of depression can help with identifying symptoms and seeking appropriate treatment. It is important to remember that depression is treatable, and seeking help is a brave step towards healing and recovery.

Chapter 2: Recognizing Depression

Everyone experiences sadness and low moods at some point in their lives. However, depression is more than just feeling sad. In this chapter, we will explore the signs and symptoms of depression and how to recognize them.

SUBCHAPTER 2.1: SIGNS AND SYMPTOMS

Depression can affect people in different ways, and there is no one definitive symptom. However, there are several common signs and symptoms that indicate a person may be struggling with depression. These include:

Feelings of sadness or hopelessness

People with depression often feel a deep sense of sadness or hopelessness that doesn't seem to go away. They may feel powerless to change their situation and may lose interest in activities they once enjoyed.

Lack of energy or fatigue

Depression can make even the simplest tasks feel overwhelming. People with depression may feel like they have no energy and may struggle to get out of bed in the morning.

Changes in appetite or weight

Depression can affect a person's appetite and eating patterns. Some people may lose their appetite and lose weight as a result, while others may overeat and gain weight.

Difficulty sleeping or oversleeping

Depression can disrupt a person's sleep patterns, causing them to have difficulty falling asleep or staying asleep. Alternatively, some people may oversleep as a way of escaping the world around them.

Loss of interest in activities

People with depression may lose interest in things they used to enjoy, such as hobbies, sports, or socializing with friends and family.

Feelings of worthlessness or guilt

Depression can cause people to feel as though they are a burden on their loved ones or that they are not contributing to society. These thoughts can lead to feelings of worthlessness and guilt.

SUBCHAPTER 2.2: SELF-ASSESSMENT

If you think you may be struggling with depression, it's important to seek help. One way to assess your symptoms is to take a depression screening test. These tests are available online and can help you determine if you're experiencing depression symptoms. Remember, diagnosing depression is not a self-diagnosis process and getting an expert opinion is always recommended.

CHAPTER 2: RECOGNIZING DEPRESSION

Subchapter 2.1: Signs and Symptoms

Depression can be a difficult condition to identify, as many of the symptoms can be attributed to other causes or simply dismissed as normal ups and downs of life. However, recognizing the signs and symptoms of depression is crucial for starting the path to recovery. Here are some common red flags to look for:

Feeling Sad or Hopeless

One of the most common symptoms of depression is feelings of persistent sadness or hopelessness. This is often accompanied by an overall lack of enjoyment in activities that previously brought pleasure.

Changes in Appetite and Sleep Patterns

Depression can also lead to changes in appetite and sleep patterns. This can manifest as either a loss of appetite and trouble sleeping or increased appetite and excessive sleep.

Fatigue and Decreased Energy

Feeling fatigued and lacking energy is another common sign of depression. This can make even simple tasks seem overwhelming and leave an individual feeling disengaged from the world around them.

Irritability and Anger

Depression can also cause irritability and anger, even over small issues. This can strain relationships and make it harder to form new connections.

Physical Discomfort

Physical symptoms such as headaches, stomachaches, and muscle pain are also common signs of depression. These symptoms can be difficult to attribute to depression and may often be misdiagnosed as an unrelated ailment. If you or someone you know is experiencing any of these symptoms, it is important to seek professional help. Depression is a treatable condition, and with the right support, it is possible to overcome it. In the next subchapter, we will explore how to conduct a self-assessment to determine if depression may be present.

SUBCHAPTER 2.2: SELF-ASSESSMENT

Recognizing the symptoms of depression is the first step toward overcoming it. However, it is not always easy to know when you are experiencing depression, especially if you have never dealt with it before. One helpful method for identifying potential depression is through self-assessment. Self-assessment involves taking a step back and honestly evaluating your own thoughts, feelings, and behaviors. This can be a useful tool for identifying patterns or changes that might indicate the presence of depression. You can start by asking yourself a few questions such as: - Do I feel more sad, irritable, or hopeless than usual? - Have I lost interest in activities that used to bring me joy? - Am I having trouble sleeping or am I sleeping too much? - Am I experiencing changes in my appetite, either overeating or not eating enough? - Do I feel tired or lacking in energy most days? - Have I noticed changes in my ability to concentrate or remember things? - Have I had thoughts of self-harm or suicide? Answering these questions can give you a sense of whether you are experiencing depression. Keep in mind that depression can manifest differently in different people, so it is important to be honest with yourself about your experiences. If you find that you are experiencing several of the symptoms listed above, it may be time to seek support from a mental health professional. Depression is a treatable condition, and there are many effective treatments available. The first step is often simply acknowledging that something is not right and taking action to address it. Don't hesitate to reach out for help if you need it.

Chapter 3: Overcoming Stigma

Stigma surrounding depression is a major contributor to the challenges faced by those who suffer from the condition. The fear of being stigmatized can prevent individuals from seeking help, leading to prolonged suffering and potentially dangerous outcomes. In this chapter, we will explore some of the common misconceptions surrounding depression and provide guidance on how to seek support and overcome the stigma associated with the condition.

SUBCHAPTER 3.1: COMMON MISCONCEPTIONS

Depression is a complex condition that is often misunderstood by those who do not experience it. Misconceptions surrounding depression can come from a variety of sources, including media portrayals and societal beliefs. Below are some of the most common misconceptions surrounding depression:

Misconception #1: Depression is a choice

One of the most damaging misconceptions surrounding depression is the belief that individuals can simply choose to "snap out of it." Depression is not a choice, and individuals who suffer from it need support and understanding from those around them.

Misconception #2: Depression is a weakness

Depression is not a weakness. It is a medical condition that requires treatment, just like any other illness. Those who suffer from depression should be treated with compassion and understanding, not judgment.

Misconception #3: Depression only affects certain types of people

Depression can affect anyone, regardless of their age, gender, or social status. It is important not to make assumptions about who may or may not be suffering from the condition.

SUBCHAPTER 3.2: SEEKING SUPPORT

Overcoming the stigma associated with depression often involves seeking support from friends, family, or mental health professionals. Below are some steps to help individuals seeking support:

Step 1: Educate yourself

Before seeking support, it may be helpful to educate yourself about depression and the various treatment options available. This can help you better understand what you or someone you know may be experiencing and the best ways to provide support.

Step 2: Reach out to others

Opening up about depression can be difficult, but it is an important step in overcoming the stigma associated with the condition. Talking with close friends or family members can provide a much-needed support system and help break down the stigma surrounding depression.

Step 3: Seek professional help

While talking with friends and family can be helpful, seeking professional help is often necessary for individuals suffering from depression. Mental health professionals can provide diagnosis and treatment options to help individuals overcome the condition and the stigma associated with it.

Step 4: Join a support group

Support groups can be a valuable resource for individuals suffering from depression. Joining a support group can provide a sense of community and help individuals realize they are not alone in their struggles.

Step 5: Be patient and persistent

Overcoming the stigma associated with depression takes time, patience, and persistence. It is important to remember that recovery is a process and not a quick fix. It is okay to struggle along the way, but seeking support and continuing treatment can help individuals overcome the stigma and thrive after depression. In conclusion, overcoming the stigma associated with depression is a challenging but important process. Educating oneself about the condition, reaching out for support, and seeking professional help can all help individuals confront and overcome the stigma surrounding depression. With persistence and patience, individuals can thrive after depression and live a healthy, fulfilling life.

COMMON MISCONCEPTIONS

There are many misconceptions surrounding depression that can make it difficult for people to seek help or understand what is happening to them. Here are some of the most common myths and the truth behind them:

Myth 1: Depression is just sadness

Depression is a serious mental health condition that affects more than just your mood. While it can cause feelings of sadness, it can also cause physical symptoms like fatigue and difficulty sleeping. Depression can also affect your ability to concentrate and make decisions, and it can lead to changes in appetite and weight.

Myth 2: Depression is a sign of weakness

Depression is not a sign of weakness, and it is not something that you can just "snap out of." Depression is a real illness that requires treatment, just like diabetes or heart disease. People with depression are not weak, and they are not to blame for their condition.

Myth 3: Depression is rare

Depression is actually very common, with an estimated 264 million people worldwide experiencing the condition. In fact, it is one of the leading causes of disability worldwide. Anyone can experience depression, regardless of their age, gender, race, or socioeconomic status.

Myth 4: Antidepressants are addictive

Antidepressants are not addictive, and they do not cause the same type of dependence as drugs like opioids or benzodiazepines. While some people may experience withdrawal symptoms if they stop taking their medication abruptly, these symptoms are usually mild and go away quickly.

Myth 5: Talking about depression only makes it worse

Talking about your depression can actually be very helpful in managing your symptoms and finding the right treatment. Keeping your feelings bottled up can make your depression worse, and it can make it harder to reach out for help. Talking to a therapist or a trusted friend or family member can help you feel less alone and more hopeful about the future. Remember, depression is a real illness that requires treatment. Don't let these misconceptions prevent you from getting the help you need.

Beating the Blues: Overcoming the Stigma of Depression

CHAPTER 3: OVERCOMING STIGMA

Subchapter 3.2: Seeking Support

Facing depression alone can be a challenging and overwhelming experience. It's essential to find support from family, friends, and healthcare professionals who can offer encouragement, compassion, and guidance to help you overcome depression. There are various types of support available for individuals suffering from depression. Seeking support can be daunting, but it is the first and most crucial step towards starting your road to recovery. Here are some support resources:

Family and Friends

Family and friends can be an excellent source of support when you're struggling with depression. It's essential to communicate with them and let them know what you're going through. Be honest and open about your feelings, and don't be afraid to ask for help. Talking to your loved ones can help you feel less isolated and alone. They can offer you moral support, encouragement, and help you with daily activities that you find challenging. Let them know what they can do to support you, whether it be listening without judgment, helping you with chores, or driving you to doctor's appointments.

Support Groups

Joining a support group can be an excellent way to connect with others who are going through the same or similar experiences. Support groups offer a safe and non-judgmental environment for individuals to share their stories and feelings. Support groups can help you feel less alone and provide you with a sense of community. You can learn coping strategies from group members that have helped them through depression as well as receive guidance and encouragement.

Healthcare Professionals

Healthcare professionals provide medical care and support to individuals with depression. These professionals include psychiatrists, psychologists, therapists, and counselors. They can offer treatment options, such as medication, therapy, and counseling. It's essential to find a healthcare professional that you feel comfortable with and can trust. They can help you develop a treatment plan, monitor your progress, and provide you with additional support. Conclusion: Seeking support is a vital part of overcoming depression. It's essential to understand that you don't have to face depression alone. There are various types of support available, including family and friends, support groups, and healthcare professionals. Remember to be kind to yourself and take the first step towards seeking the support you need and deserve.

Chapter 4: Coping Strategies

Coping strategies play an essential role in managing and overcoming depression. Depression can make things feel overwhelming and even impossible, but with the right tools, you can cope with your feelings and begin to feel better. In this chapter, we'll discuss various coping strategies that you can use to manage your depression.

SUBCHAPTER 4.1: SELF-CARE

Self-care involves engaging in activities that can improve your mental, emotional, and physical well-being. When you're experiencing depression, it's essential to prioritize self-care. Here are some self-care strategies to consider:

1. Get enough sleep

One of the essential aspects of self-care is getting enough sleep. Sleep is crucial for overall health and can help improve your mood and energy levels.

2. Eat a healthy diet

Eating a healthy diet can also help improve your overall well-being. Avoiding processed foods and consuming more fresh fruits and vegetables can help improve your mood and energy levels. Additionally, avoiding caffeine and alcohol can also help improve your overall mental health.

3. Engage in physical activity

Physical activity has been shown to help with depression symptoms. Even light exercise, such as walking or yoga, can help improve your mood and energy levels.

SUBCHAPTER 4.2: PROFESSIONAL TREATMENT OPTIONS

In addition to self-care strategies, there are also professional treatment options available to help individuals cope with depression. Here are some of the most common forms of professional treatment:

1. Therapy

Therapy, or counseling, involves talking to a mental health professional to address your depression symptoms. Therapy can help you work through issues and learn coping mechanisms to manage your depression.

2. Medication

Medication can also be helpful for treating depression. Antidepressants are commonly prescribed to individuals with depression and can help improve mood and energy levels.

3. Support groups

Support groups involve meeting with others who are experiencing similar symptoms to discuss and share experiences. Support groups can be helpful for individuals who feel isolated or who may not have access to therapy. In conclusion, coping strategies are essential for managing depression. Whether it's engaging in self-care strategies or seeking professional treatment, there are many ways to cope with your symptoms and begin to feel better. Remember, depression is a treatable condition, and with the right tools and support, you can overcome it.

SUBCHAPTER 4.1: SELF-CARE

Taking care of yourself is a crucial part of managing depression. Self-care involves intentionally doing things that make you feel better physically, mentally, and emotionally. It is not a selfish act, but rather a necessary step to improve your well-being.

Physical Self-Care

Physical self-care involves taking care of your body. This includes exercising regularly, eating healthy foods, and getting enough sleep. Exercise has been proven to reduce symptoms of depression by increasing endorphins, which are feel-good chemicals in the brain. Eating a healthy diet can also improve your mood and energy level. Lastly, getting enough sleep is vital for both physical and emotional health.

Mental Self-Care

Mental self-care involves taking care of your mind. This includes engaging in activities that give you pleasure, such as hobbies or reading. It also involves managing stress through practices such as mindfulness, meditation, or deep breathing exercises. Practicing gratitude and positive self-talk can also help improve your mental health.

Emotional Self-Care

Emotional self-care involves taking care of your emotions. This includes being aware of your feelings, expressing them in a healthy way, and seeking support when needed. It is important to be kind and compassionate to yourself, and to avoid self-criticism. Cultivating healthy relationships and setting boundaries can also help improve your emotional well-being.

Self-Care Tips

Here are some self-care tips to get you started: - Take time for yourself each day to engage in an activity you enjoy. - Practice good hygiene, like showering and brushing your teeth regularly. - Set aside time to exercise each day, even if it's just a short walk. - Try to eat a healthy, balanced diet. - Get enough sleep each night (7-9 hours is recommended for adults). - Practice mindfulness or meditation as a daily routine. - Engage in relaxation techniques like deep breathing exercises. - Reach out to friends or family for support when needed. - Practice positive self-talk and gratitude daily. Remember that self-care is not a one-time event, but rather a consistent effort to take care of yourself. By prioritizing self-care, you can improve your mood and overall well-being.

Beating the Blues: Overcoming the Stigma of Depression

CHAPTER 4: COPING STRATEGIES

Subchapter 4.2: Professional Treatment Options

If you're struggling with depression, seeking professional help can significantly improve your chances of recovery. While self-help techniques and support from friends and family can be helpful, they might not be enough to address the root causes of depression. However, with the right professional support, you can learn how to manage your symptoms and develop coping skills to lead a healthy and fulfilling life. Here are some professional treatment options for depression:

Medication:

Antidepressants are commonly prescribed to help manage depression. These medications work by altering the levels of chemicals in the brain that affect mood. It is important to work closely with your healthcare provider to find the right medication, dosage, and length of treatment. While medication can be helpful, it's important to remember that it may not work for everyone, and it should always be combined with other forms of treatment, such as therapy and lifestyle changes.

Therapy:

Various types of therapy can be helpful in treating depression. Cognitive-behavioral therapy, or CBT, is a type of therapy that focuses on changing negative thought patterns that contribute to depression. It helps you identify and change negative thoughts and beliefs, and develop a more positive outlook. Another type of therapy that can be helpful is interpersonal therapy. This form of therapy focuses on improving communication and relationship skills, and can be particularly helpful for people struggling with depression related to relationship problems.

Electroconvulsive Therapy (ECT):

Electroconvulsive therapy (ECT) is a medical treatment for severe depression. It involves passing a small electric current through the brain in order to trigger a seizure. While it might sound scary, ECT is generally safe, and a highly effective treatment for certain forms of depression. It is typically reserved for people with severe, treatment-resistant depression.

Transcranial Magnetic Stimulation (TMS):

Transcranial magnetic stimulation (TMS) is a procedure that uses magnetic fields to stimulate nerve cells in the brain. It is a relatively new treatment for depression, and while it may not work for everyone, it can be an effective treatment option for some people, especially those who have not benefited from traditional medication or therapy. TMS is typically an outpatient procedure and is performed in a physician's office. Remember, everyone is different, and what works for one person might not work for another. If you're struggling with depression, it's important to work with a healthcare professional to find the right treatment plan for you. Don't be afraid to reach out for help; seeking treatment is a sign of strength.

Chapter 5: Building a Support System

At times when we feel low, it can be challenging to pull ourselves together. Reaching out for help is not a sign of weakness, but rather a sign of strength. Building a support system can provide the necessary resources and encouragement to overcome depression. In this chapter, we will explore various aspects of creating a support network.

SUBCHAPTER 5.1: COMMUNICATION SKILLS

Effective communication skills play an important role in building a support network. People need to understand what type of support you need in order to provide it. Therefore, it is essential to communicate your emotions and thoughts with your loved ones. It is important to find individuals who can listen to you without judgment and criticism. Try to express your feelings and thoughts in an assertive manner rather than an aggressive or passive tone. Assertive communication emphasizes respect for your own opinions and the needs of others. On the other hand, aggressive communication focuses on only your needs and feelings, whereas passive communication disregards them altogether. Active listening is also a crucial aspect of communication. When a loved one is speaking to you, try to put aside your thoughts and listen actively to what they are saying. Provide them with your complete attention and affirm their emotions and thoughts.

SUBCHAPTER 5.2: RELATIONSHIPS AND BOUNDARIES

It is important to developing healthy relationships where both parties understand each other's boundaries. Boundaries can be physical or emotional and are necessary for the maintenance of a healthy relationship. If someone in your life is causing unnecessary stress or toxic emotions, you need to set clear boundaries with them. Setting boundaries does not mean you have to cut off ties completely but rather limit your interactions with the person. It is essential to prioritize your mental health and wellbeing above a relationship that causes unnecessary emotional distress. On the other hand, healthy relationships are built on mutual respect, trust, and communication. Surrounding yourself with loving, positive people who encourage and uplift you can be a huge boost for your mental health.

CONCLUSION

Beating the Blues: Overcoming the Stigma of Depression

CHAPTER 5: BUILDING A SUPPORT SYSTEM

Subchapter 5.1: Communication Skills

Effective communication is key to building a strong support system when dealing with depression. Depression can make it difficult to communicate your needs and feelings clearly, but with some practice, you can develop the skills necessary to express yourself. The first step in effective communication is learning to listen actively. Active listening means paying attention to what the other person is saying and acknowledging their feelings. When you actively listen, you are showing the other person that you care about what they are saying, which can help build trust and open up lines of communication. It's also essential to express yourself honestly and directly. Be clear about what you need and how you are feeling. Use "I" statements to take ownership of your thoughts and feelings rather than placing blame on others. For example, saying "I feel like my depression is taking over my life" communicates your feelings more effectively than saying "You're making me depressed." Another crucial aspect of communication is learning to communicate boundaries effectively. It's okay to say "no" to things that you don't have the energy or interest in doing. Communicating boundaries can help reduce stress and prevent feelings of overwhelm or burnout. Finally, don't be afraid to ask for help. It can be challenging to ask for help when dealing with depression, but it's important to remember that it's okay to not be okay. Reach out to family, friends, or mental health professionals for support and guidance. In conclusion, effective communication is key to building a strong support system when dealing with depression. Learning to listen actively, express yourself honestly and directly, communicate boundaries effectively, and ask for help when needed can all help improve your communication skills and ultimately, your mental well-being.

CHAPTER 5: BUILDING A SUPPORT SYSTEM

Subchapter 5.2: Relationships and Boundaries

When dealing with depression, having a strong support system can make all the difference in your recovery. While receiving help from professionals and support groups is crucial, building healthy relationships with family and friends is also an important aspect of building a support system. It's important to remember that not everyone will understand what you're going through, and that's okay. The key is to surround yourself with people who acknowledge your struggles and are willing to listen and support you without judgment. When building relationships, it's also important to set boundaries. This means being clear about what you need and what you don't need from others. It's okay to say "no" to things that don't serve your mental health and well-being. Here are a few tips on how to build healthy relationships and set boundaries: 1. Communicate openly: When you're feeling overwhelmed or stressed, share your feelings with your loved ones. By being honest and open, you'll build trust and create a space for them to support you. 2. Be clear about what you need: If you need space or time alone, communicate that to the people in your life. Explain that it's not personal, but that you're prioritizing your mental health. 3. Practice self-care: Taking care of yourself is the foundation of building healthy relationships. Make sure you're taking time for yourself and doing things that bring you joy and relaxation. 4. Be patient: It's important to remember that building strong relationships takes time. Allow yourself and your loved ones patience and understanding as you navigate this journey together. Remember, building healthy relationships is a two-way street. Be open to giving and receiving support, and always be kind and compassionate with yourself and those around you. By creating a strong support system built on trust and understanding, you'll have a solid foundation for overcoming the stigma of depression.

Chapter 6: Maintaining a Healthy Mindset

After overcoming depression, it is crucial to maintain a healthy mindset and prevent relapse. Maintaining a healthy mindset requires a conscious effort every day. Here are some techniques that can be helpful in maintaining a healthy mindset.

SUBCHAPTER 6.1: MINDFULNESS TECHNIQUES

Mindfulness is a technique that can help you improve your mental wellbeing. Mindfulness is the process of paying attention to your thoughts, emotions, and physical sensations in a non-judgmental way. Mindfulness can be practiced through meditation, breathing exercises, and other techniques. Here are some mindfulness techniques that can help you maintain a healthy mindset.

Body Scan Meditation

Body scan meditation is a form of meditation that involves scanning your body from head to toe. It helps you become aware of the sensations in your body and brings your attention to the present moment. To practice body scan meditation, find a quiet place to sit or lie down, close your eyes, and start scanning your body from your head to your toes. Observe any sensations or feelings that you may experience without judgement.

Breathing Exercises

Breathing exercises are a quick and easy way to calm your mind and reduce stress. One breathing exercise that can be helpful is the 4-7-8 breathing technique. To practice this technique, inhale for 4 seconds, hold your breath for 7 seconds, and exhale for 8 seconds. Repeat this exercise for several minutes until you feel calm and relaxed.

SUBCHAPTER 6.2: POSITIVE PSYCHOLOGY PRINCIPLES

Positive psychology is a branch of psychology that focuses on what makes people happy and fulfilled. Positive psychology principles can help you maintain a healthy mindset by fostering positive emotions, thoughts, and behaviors. Here are some positive psychology principles that can help you maintain a healthy mindset.

Gratitude Practice

Gratitude is a powerful emotion that can help you maintain a positive mindset. Practicing gratitude involves focusing on the things you are thankful for in your life. You can practice gratitude by keeping a gratitude journal, where you write down three things you are thankful for each day. Another way to practice gratitude is to express your gratitude to others through a thank-you note or verbal expression.

Positive Affirmations

Positive affirmations are statements that you repeat to yourself to encourage positive thinking and behavior. Positive affirmations can help you develop a positive mindset by cultivating self-confidence and self-belief. Examples of positive affirmations include "I am capable and strong," "I am worthy of love and respect," and "I am grateful for my life and everything in it." Maintaining a healthy mindset is crucial in preventing depression relapse. By practicing mindfulness techniques and positive psychology principles, you can cultivate a healthy mindset and improve your overall wellbeing. Remember to practice these techniques regularly and seek professional support if needed.

CHAPTER 6: MAINTAINING A HEALTHY MINDSET

Subchapter 6.1: Mindfulness Techniques

Living in today's fast-paced world, it's easy to get caught up in the stresses of daily life. Work, school, and personal responsibilities can leave little time for relaxation and self-reflection. However, taking the time to practice mindfulness can greatly improve our mental and emotional wellbeing. Mindfulness is the practice of being present in the current moment and fully engaged in one's surroundings. It's about observing and accepting our thoughts and feelings without judgment. With mindfulness, we can become more aware of our own mental processes and learn how to manage negative thoughts and emotions. One of the most popular and effective mindfulness techniques is meditation. This involves sitting comfortably in a quiet place and focusing on your breath. As thoughts enter your mind, you acknowledge them but then return your focus to your breath. Over time, meditation can help calm the mind, reduce stress, and improve overall mood. Another way to practice mindfulness is to pay attention to your senses. This involves fully experiencing the sights, sounds, smells, flavors, and textures of your surroundings. By engaging your senses in this way, you can connect with the present moment and feel more grounded. Mindfulness can also be incorporated into daily activities such as exercise, cooking, or even showering. By focusing on the task at hand and fully immersing yourself in the experience, you can cultivate a sense of mindfulness and relaxation. In conclusion, mindfulness techniques such as meditation, sensory awareness, and fully engaging in daily activities can greatly improve our mental and emotional health. By practicing mindfulness, we can learn to manage stress, reduce negative thoughts and emotions, and cultivate a sense of peace and wellbeing.

SUBCHAPTER 6.2: POSITIVE PSYCHOLOGY PRINCIPLES

Positive psychology is a relatively new branch of psychology that seeks to focus on mental wellness and resiliency, rather than solely on diagnosing and treating problems. Instead of only looking at what may be causing an individual's depression, positive psychology also concentrates on what is working well in their lives and how those strengths can be maximized to improve their overall well-being. So, what are some of the principles of positive psychology that can be beneficial for people struggling with depression?

Cultivating Gratitude

One of the primary ways to increase overall happiness and promote mental wellness is to cultivate gratitude. This means taking the time to notice and appreciate the positive things in your life, no matter how small they may seem. This practice can help you shift your focus away from negative thoughts and experiences, and instead, focus on the blessings and opportunities that are present in your life. There are several ways to cultivate gratitude in your life. You could start by keeping a daily journal in which you write down a few things you are grateful for each day, or you could make it a habit to express gratitude to others as often as possible.

Fostering Positive Relationships

Positive relationships are an essential part of overall well-being. People who have strong, supportive relationships with friends, family, and romantic partners are typically happier, healthier, and more resilient than those who do not. If you are struggling with depression, it can be tough to put yourself out there and build new relationships. Still, it is essential to remember that relationships take time and effort to grow. You could consider joining a club or group centered around one of your interests, where you could meet like-minded individuals and form new connections.

Cultivating Optimism

Optimism is the belief that good things will happen in the future, even if the present may feel challenging. Cultivating optimism can help individuals with depression cope better with stress, persevere through difficult times, and see the good in their lives. It can be challenging to feel optimistic when you are experiencing depression, but small habits can help cultivate this mindset. Doing things you love, such as hobbies or spending time with loved ones, can help shift your focus toward more hopeful and positive feelings. Overall, positive psychology principles can be a helpful addition to any depression treatment plan. By focusing on building relationships, cultivating gratitude, and fostering optimism, individuals can improve their overall well-being and resilience.

Chapter 7: Thriving After Depression

Depression can consume a person's life, but it doesn't have to define it. Recovery is a process, and it takes time, effort, and a significant amount of resilience. The path to thriving after depression may seem daunting, but it is entirely achievable.

SUBCHAPTER 7.1: MOVING FORWARD

Moving forward after depression isn't about pretending it never happened. It's about processing what you've been through and using it as an opportunity for growth. There are several ways to do this on your own, but it's also essential to seek support when you need it. One great way to start is by setting small goals that can help you cultivate new experiences. Maybe it's trying a new hobby, taking a class, or volunteering. By doing things that help you feel good about yourself and the world around you, you can start to create a new narrative in your life. Another effective way to move forward is by exploring the ways depression has impacted your values, priorities, and worldview. Depression can be a period of inner growth, so it's worth asking yourself what it has taught you about the things that matter most to you. You might find that you have a renewed appreciation for your relationships, a new career goal, or even a more solidified sense of self.

SUBCHAPTER 7.2: EMBRACING RESILIENCE

Resilience is the ability to bounce back from adversity, and it is essential to thriving after depression. Nobody is immune to life's challenges, but building resilience allows you to weather them with more grace and come out stronger on the other side. One way to build resilience is by practicing self-care regularly. You've likely heard of the basics: exercise, nutrition, sleep, and stress management. But self-care can also mean engaging in activities that bring you joy, cultivating positive relationships, and practicing self-compassion. Another important way to embrace resilience is by reframing your view of setbacks. Instead of seeing them as failures, view them as opportunities for growth. This means stepping back, reflecting on what you learned, and using that knowledge to keep moving forward.

Maintaining Hope

Hope is the belief that things will get better, and it is crucial for thriving after depression. By maintaining hope, you can avoid falling back into old patterns and thought patterns that kept you trapped in depression in the first place. Remember that recovery is not a linear process, and setbacks are a part of the journey. The important thing is to stay committed to your recovery and trust that you are moving in the right direction. By continuing to seek support, engaging in self-care, and embracing resilience, you can not only overcome depression but also thrive in your life beyond it.

In Conclusion

Thriving after depression is possible. It takes hard work, resilience, and hope, but it is entirely achievable. If you or someone you know is struggling with depression, remember that recovery is a process, and there is no shame in seeking support. With time, patience, and perseverance, you can go beyond simply beating the blues and create a joyful, fulfilling life.

SUBCHAPTER 7.1: MOVING FORWARD

Moving forward after experiencing depression can be a daunting task. It's important to remember that recovery is not a linear process, and there may be setbacks along the way. However, with dedication and perseverance, it is possible to not only recover but also thrive. It's important to take an active role in your recovery and make small, achievable goals for yourself. Celebrating these milestones can help you stay motivated and on track. Surrounding yourself with a positive support system can also be helpful during this time. It's important to continue practicing self-care, as depression can leave you feeling depleted. Incorporating daily exercise, a healthy diet, and hobbies that bring you joy can also help improve your overall well-being. Seeking professional support, such as therapy or medication, can also be an integral part of moving forward. It's important to work with a licensed mental health professional to determine the best course of treatment for you. Accepting and learning from past experiences can also be a key part of moving forward. It's important to identify any patterns or triggers that may have contributed to your depression and take steps to avoid or manage them in the future. Remember, moving forward is a process, and it's important to be patient and kind to yourself along the way. You have the strength and resilience to overcome depression and create a fulfilling life for yourself.